MW01600257

THE INTEGRATED MAN

A Handbook For The Recovering Nice Guy

SIDHARTH AGARWAL

WILDMANCOACHING.COM

First Edition: 2023
Published by Sidharth Agarwal
(wildmancoaching.com)

Disclaimer

Although you may find the information, principles, applications, and assignments in this book to be useful, they are presented with the understanding that the author is not engaged, or intending to engage, in providing specific medical, psychological, emotional, or sexual advice. Nor is anything in this book intended to be a diagnosis, prescription, recommendation, or cure for any specific kind of medical, psychological, emotional, or sexual problem. Each person has unique needs, and this book cannot take these individual differences into account. Each person should engage in a program of treatment, prevention, cure, and/or general health only in consultation with licensed, qualified physicians, therapists, and/or other competent professionals.

Acknowledgment

There is a unique phenomenon about the book *"No More Mr. Nice Guy: A Proven Plan for Getting What You Want in Love, Sex, and Life"* by Dr. Robert Glover that I have never seen with any other book. It is this: I have met hundreds of men who couldn't help but feel that the author was describing their experiences and struggles perfectly. They are amazed at how accurately Dr. Glover captured their thoughts and feelings, and they can't help but feel that Dr. Glover wrote the book specifically for them. This is also how I felt when I first read Dr. Glover's book many years ago when trying to get my life together after a painful divorce. I hated Dr. Glover for somehow knowing my deepest, darkest secrets, and I loved him for laying out a proven plan to help me get over my struggles as a nice guy.

This is testimony to the genius of Dr. Glover and the continued importance and relevance of his seminal work, *No More Mr. Nice Guy*. I am honored to call him a mentor and to be one of his certified coaches. Dr. Glover's book continues to be one of the essential resources for male initiation for countless men. (More on male initiation later in the introduction.)

Over time, men began to reach out to me for coaching to get support in recovering from their *Nice Guy Syndrome*. Over some months, I saw these men transform from scared nice guys to confident, integrated men. It has been an enriching journey for me to be able to help these men step into their greatness.

But here's another thing about nice guys: they tend to be bad finishers. They rarely finish what they often start with enthusiasm, including personal development projects, jobs, relationships, and even books. While men would often come to me after reading the first few chapters of *No More Mr. Nice Guy*, I noticed that most rarely got to the end of the book. I'd often hear some version of this sentence, "I began reading the book two (or four or five) years back, and I think I really need to take some action."

To help my coaching clients benefit from the wealth of valuable information in *No More Mr. Nice Guy*, I began summarizing key concepts from the book and incorporating insights and tools from my journey of "Nice Guy" recovery. I included these summaries in a private newsletter to my clients, and that's how this handbook was born.

I am immensely thankful to Dr. Robert Glover for the profound impact he has had on my life and the lives of many others. His pioneering work laid the foundation for this book, and I am deeply indebted to him. This guide is dedicated to all the individuals who identify as Nice Guys who have been struggling and searching for answers. I sincerely hope that the information and strategies presented in this book will assist you in finding your greatness.

Foreword by Dr. Robert Glover

It's 3:30 in the afternoon where I am in the US Central time zone when I get notification of a text message. It's from Sid. He's just sent me an elaborate diagram or spreadsheet based on a subject we talked about earlier in the day. As I marvel at the clarity of thinking and creative design he has put into the page in front of me, a thought crosses my mind; "What the hell time is it in Pune, India?

I check the time zone app on my phone, and pretty much as I thought, it's 2:00 a.m. where Sid is.

When he and I talked earlier in the day about the information he has now beautifully synthesized and organized into the document I'm looking at on my computer screen, it was probably around

10:00 PM his time – a time when most folks would be winding down and ready to turn out the lights. But four hours later, there is this work of art in my inbox.

That's Sidharth.

My first connection with Sid was in early 2019, when he contacted me about coming to my No More Mr. Nice Guy Coach Certification workshop in Seattle. Over the years, several men had come from some pretty distant geographical locales to join me in Seattle or Puerto Vallarta, where I hold most of my workshops, but Pune, India, seemed to top them all.

Upon meeting Sid in Seattle, it didn't take long for me to realize that underneath a humble, unassuming exterior (he is not only Indian, but he's also a Buddhist), was a razor sharp mind and an enthusiastic demeanor.

Since then, I've discovered how deep this intellect and enthusiasm run – especially in terms of doing men's work.

Every time I put out a notice to my certified coaches seeking volunteers to help me with an online workshop or program, Sid is one of the first to respond and volunteer (sometimes I wonder if he ever sleeps). Not only does he volunteer, but he also lets me know that he is available to help out in any way he can – and he means it.

Not only is Sid passionate about helping men around the world shed the Nice Guy Syndrome and become Integrated Men, but he is also pretty much single-handedly working to bring the Mankind Project to the men of India. He's a fucking machine.

So, when Sid asked me if I could look over the "handbook" he had written as a supplement to my book, No More Mr. Nice Guy (Running Press, 2003), I thought, "Well, that's the least I could do."

As I began to read the pages of the book you now have in your hand, I kept thinking, "Yeah, he explained that well," and "He really did a good job of capturing how my message on this concept has evolved since I wrote NMMNG over 25 years ago."

For me, that's the beauty of The Integrated Man; it builds on the concepts I presented in No More Mr. Nice Guy over two decades ago but also further refines and updates them based on what I teach today.

Plus, this book contains subjects I now teach that weren't even on my radar back in 2003, when NMMNG was published.

The Integrated Man brings No More Mr. Nice Guy into the 2020s.

Subjects that Sid updates and clarifies in The

Integrated Man include the concept of covert contracts, abandonment anxiety, and toxic shame —the one-two-punch of the Nice Guy Syndrome —the need for masculine initiation, and boundaries.

Other topics that now show up in my courses, workshops, and more recent books that were not presented in No More Mr. Nice Guy that Sid includes in The Integrated Man include, self-soothing, abundance thinking, rejection sensitivity, the four traits of the Integrated Man, and self-limiting beliefs.

Woven throughout this compact handbook are Sid's suggestions for ways the reader (you) can apply the principles presented.

Just like those amazing diagrams and spreadsheets that Sid creates when he really should be sleeping, he has created a concise, elegant, and impressive update of the NMMNG message.

I can't recommend this book highly enough. It is so much more than just a handbook; it is a deep-dive into complex concepts in a quick and easy read – and that's impressive. But hey, that's Sidharth.

Robert A. Glover, Ph.D.
Puerto Vallarta, Mexico
26 April 2023

Table Of Contents

Introduction

The Absence of Male Initiation

In many ways, the prevalence of the *Nice Guy Syndrome* among modern men is a manifestation of a lack of male initiation. So, let's start with a history lesson about male initiation.

Male initiation is a profound rite of passage that has captivated the human imagination for centuries. It is a ceremony that marks the transition from boyhood to manhood and is a powerful symbol of the journey from adolescence to adulthood.

Historically, the male initiation ceremony is often associated with traditional and indigenous cultures. For example, many African cultures have practiced male initiation ceremonies for centuries. In the Xhosa culture of South Africa, for example, young men undergo a rite of passage known as the *ulwaluko*, which involves instruction in the responsibilities and duties of adulthood. In some Polynesian cultures, young men were expected to participate in a rite of passage known as the "mauli," which involved tattooing and training in martial arts.

A typical male initiation involved a series of rituals and ceremonies designed to test the initiate's strength, endurance, and courage. These rituals often included physical challenges such as hunting, warfare, endurance tests, and spiritual and cultural teachings. Through these challenges, young men demonstrated their readiness to assume the responsibilities and duties of adulthood and prove their worthiness as full-fledged community members.

The role of older men in organizing a male initiation was crucial. They were responsible for passing on the cultural traditions and values of the community to the next generation, and they were the guardians of the knowledge and wisdom imparted during the initiation ceremony. They guided and mentored the young men and ultimately decided when a boy was ready to become a man.

Initiation served as a powerful symbol of the continuity and preservation of the community. It was a way of reinforcing social cohesion and creating a sense of shared identity among its members. It was a way of passing on the cultural heritage and wisdom of the ancestors to the next generation, ensuring that the community would continue to thrive and flourish for many generations to come.

These male initiation ceremonies were essential for the socialization and education of young men.

They often involved teachings about responsibility, duty, and morality and were intended to prepare young men for adulthood and their roles as leaders and protectors within the community.

Modern society has largely abandoned traditional initiation rituals, leading to many negative impacts. Some of the potential adverse effects include:

- Lack of guidance and mentorship: Traditional initiation rituals involved guidance and mentorship from older men, who passed on their knowledge, wisdom, and experience to the next generation. Without these rituals, young men do not have the same level of guidance and mentorship, which can lead to confusion and uncertainty as they navigate adulthood.

- Lack of direction and purpose: Initiation rituals provided a sense of direction and purpose for young men as they were initiated into the roles and responsibilities of adulthood. These rituals are necessary for young men to have the same sense of purpose and struggle to find direction and meaning in their lives.

- Loss of cultural identity: With initiation rituals, young men have a different sense of connection to their cultural heritage and feel more firmly rooted in their community. Initiation rituals often serve as a way of creating a sense of shared identity among community members. These rituals are necessary for young men to have more social cohesion and a stronger sense of community.

- Lack of a rite of passage: Initiation rituals were a rite of passage, marking the transition from adolescence to adulthood. Without these rituals, the transition from boyhood to manhood is less meaningful, and young men do not have the same sense of accomplishment or pride in their new status as adult members of the community.

As modern men, we are in a unique and challenging position. The absence of traditional initiation rituals has left us without a clear path to navigate the transition from boyhood to manhood. But this should not be seen as a curse but as an opportunity for self-discovery and growth.

It is a call to action, a call to take responsibility for our lives and development. It is a call to design and go through our rite of passage, which is true to our values and beliefs.

For it is not only a responsibility to ourselves but to our communities as well. We are the leaders, protectors, and providers of our families, friends, and communities. We must become the best versions of ourselves, live with integrity, and contribute positively to the world.

This is not a task to be taken lightly, but with compassion, urgency, and a profound understanding of the significance of this rite of passage. It is a journey that requires courage, determination, and self-reflection. It is a journey that is not without its challenges but is ultimately rewarding and fulfilling.

Let us not shy away from this calling. Let us embrace it and become the men we are meant to be. In doing so, we will fulfill our potential and inspire and empower those around us to do the same.

I hope this handbook is a reference resource and toolkit for recovering *Nice Guys* on the path to their initiation.

This book narrates the semi-fictional stories of three recovering Nice Guys – Ryan, Neil, and

Rowan. Through their Hero's Journey of Nice Guys' recovery, I tease out what the *Nice Guy Syndrome* is, what causes it, and some of the most reliable concepts and tools I have discovered to help my clients become *integrated men.*

Understanding the Nice Guy Syndrome

But What's Wrong With Being Nice?

That's a question I get about five times a day from potential coaching clients, friends, family, and people I have just met. Here's the deal: being nice is great. But the Nice Guys I'm talking about are frauds. They are *fraudulently nice*, that is. I know these guys. I used to be one.

You know the type: they act kind and considerate, but their motivations are selfish or manipulative. Sound familiar? It's called the *"Nice Guy Syndrome,"* when guys try to suck up to others, especially women, by being super helpful or accommodating to win their favor. But here's the thing: it's not genuine. And when their efforts aren't appreciated or don't bring the desired results, they get resentful or angry.

Fraudulent niceness causes problems in relationships because it's not real. It's just a facade to get something from the other person – love, approval, a sense of control. But since it's not based on genuine care or concern for the other person, it's not sustainable and leads to resentment, bitterness, and disillusionment. People can sense when someone is being insincerely nice, and it makes them feel manipulated or used. Trust breaks down, and so do relationships.

This behavior is especially prevalent in the dating world, where a guy will try to be extra kind and accommodating to his crush in the hopes of winning her affection. But that lack of authenticity can be a major turn-off. In the workplace, fraudulent niceness may mean sucking up to the boss or coworkers to get ahead instead of just being a hard worker and team player. In friendships, it may involve constantly agreeing with others and not standing up for yourself to avoid confrontation or to be liked.

Bottom line: fraudulent niceness doesn't work because it's not genuine. It leads to frustration and resentment for the *nice guy* and can push others further away. So let's ditch the act and get real.

Let's Meet Some Nice Guys

Let's meet three *Nice Guy*s – Ryan, Neil, and Rowan. We'll follow them throughout this book as they take their Hero's Journey from being *Nice Guys* to becoming *Integrated Men*. Although these characters are semi-fictional, in their stories you'll find reflections of yourself and men you know.

Ryan

Ryan was a classic *Nice Guy* – always going out of his way to make everyone else happy, no matter what it took. So, when he overheard his long-time crush Sara talking about her love for a rare coffee bean that could only be found at a specialty shop in the next town over, he saw it as the perfect opportunity to win her over.

"I'll be her designated driver," he thought to himself. "I'll show her how selfless and thoughtful I am." And with that, he offered to drive her to the store to buy the coffee.

Little did he know, the store was a solid hour's drive away. But Ryan didn't mind – he was on a mission. He spent hours on the round trip, even paying for the coffee himself. But despite his heroic efforts, Sara barely even noticed.

"No problem," Ryan told himself. "I'll just keep

doing favors for her, and eventually, she'll see how much I care." And so he continued to go above and beyond for Sara, even putting up with her sometimes rude or thoughtless behavior. "If I just try hard enough," he thought, "she'll eventually see how much I love her."

But the harder he tried, the more distant and uninterested Sara seemed. Ryan began to feel frustrated and resentful, but he couldn't give up. He was stuck in a cycle of trying to win Sara's affection through self-sacrifice, all the while unable to understand why she seemed to grow more and more disinterested in him.

"I'm just being a good person," he told himself. "I'm showing her that I care. I'm trying to be the best possible future partner I can be." These thoughts might have made Ryan feel better about his actions, but they also kept him from realizing that his efforts were driving him to the friendzone faster than a Formula 1 race driver.

Neil

Neil was stuck in a tough spot. He knew his wife was unfaithful, but he didn't want to cause conflict or disrupt his family. He hoped that if he just kept being the best husband he could be, his wife would eventually see the error of her ways and stop cheating.

But as the weeks and months dragged on, Neil found himself feeling more and more unhappy. He was heartbroken and devastated by his wife's infidelity, and he couldn't understand why she couldn't see how much he was hurting. Despite his attempts to be supportive and understanding, his wife showed no signs of changing her behavior.

Neil couldn't bring himself to confront his wife about the affair and was scared of being alone, trapped in a cycle of trying to be the "perfect" husband, even at the cost of his well being.

It's not uncommon for people in Neil's situation to make excuses or rationalizations for why they stay in an unhealthy or unhappy relationship. Neil told himself:

"I don't want to be alone."

"I don't want to break up my family."

"I don't want to disappoint or hurt anyone."

"I hope things will get better eventually."

"I'm afraid of change."

"I don't want to admit that my marriage is a failure."

"I don't want to give up on the person I love."

Despite his misery and frustration, Neil couldn't bring himself to confront his wife. He was caught in a problematic cycle and didn't know how to break free.

Rowan

Rowan was a *Nice Guy* at work who always tried to be helpful and cooperative. He was eager to please his colleagues and his boss and was always willing to go the extra mile to get the job done. However, his behavior often had unintended consequences.

For example, Rowan had difficulty setting boundaries and saying "no" to requests for his time and energy. As a result, he often felt overwhelmed and overworked and struggled to balance his job with his personal life. His colleagues also took advantage of his willingness to help, often assigning him additional tasks or responsibilities without considering his workload.

Rowan's lack of assertiveness and confidence also hindered his career advancement. He was hesitant to speak up for himself or to advocate for his own needs and ideas, and he often felt overshadowed by more confident and assertive colleagues. This led to frustration and resentment for Rowan, as he felt his hard work and dedication were not being recognized or appreciated.

Despite these challenges, Rowan continued to play nice at work, hoping his efforts would eventually be recognized and rewarded.

The Nice Guy's Covert Contracts

The *Nice Guy Syndrome* refers to a pattern of behavior in which a man is nice to others, particularly women, in the hopes of gaining approval and affection. These men may try to do favors for others and avoid confrontation, but their motivation is often self-serving, as they hope to be rewarded with love and acceptance. This behavior is often unhealthy and harmful, as it can lead to resentment and frustration on the part of the *nice guy* and can also be manipulative and controlling.

It is not uncommon for individuals who exhibit the *Nice Guy Syndrome* to have certain expectations or unspoken agreements, known as "covert contracts," in their relationships with others. These contracts can be subtle and unconscious. They may involve the belief that their efforts to be nice should be rewarded with love, affection, or other forms of validation. Often, many men who come to me for coaching don't even realize that they are operating with these covert contracts.

The following three fundamental covert contracts guide *Nice Guys*:

1. If I am a good guy, everyone will love and like me (and the people I desire will desire me).

2. If I meet other people's needs without them having to ask, they will fulfill my needs without me having to ask.

3. If I do everything right, I will have a smooth, problem-free life.

These three fundamental covert contracts manifest in hidden assumptions in the Nice Guy's relationships. These are:

- The "I'll be nice to you if you're nice to me" contract: This contract is based on the belief that if the *nice guy* is kind, helpful, and accommodating to others, he should receive the same treatment in return without him having to ask for what he needs.

- The "I'll do things for you if you do things for me" contract: This contract involves the idea that if the *nice guy* performs favors or goes out of his way to help others, they should repay him with gestures of appreciation or affection.

- The "I'll be there for you if you're there for me" contract: This contract is based on the belief that if the *nice guy* is supportive and available for others, he should be able to count on the same level of support and availability in return.

- The "If I do things for you, you will have sex with me" contract: This covert contract involves distorted beliefs about what makes others sexually attracted and open. The *nice guy* believes that a woman will have sex with him if he goes out of his way to do things for her.

- The "I'll be good if you're good to me" contract: This contract involves the belief that if the *nice guy* follows the rules and behaves well, he should be rewarded with love and affection.

- The "I'll be there for you no matter what" contract: This contract involves the idea that the *nice guy* will always be available and supportive, no matter the circumstances.

- The "I'll do anything for you" contract: This contract involves the belief that the *nice guy* will go to great lengths to please others, even if it means sacrificing his own needs or desires.

- The "I'll change for you" contract: This contract involves the belief that the *nice guy* will modify his behavior or personality in order to gain the approval and affection of others.

- The "I'll put up with anything" contract: This contract involves the idea that the *nice guy* will endure mistreatment or abuse in the hopes of being loved or accepted.

- The "I'll always be there for you" contract: This contract involves the belief that the *nice guy* will always be available and supportive, even if it becomes emotionally or physically draining.

- The "I'll do anything to win your love" contract: This contract involves the belief that the *nice guy* will go to great lengths to win the affection of others, even if it means compromising his values or sense of self.

- The "I'll be your friend if you'll be my friend" contract: This contract is based on the belief that if the *nice guy* is a good friend to someone, he should be able to expect the same level of friendship in return.

- The "I'll support you if you support me" contract: This contract involves the idea that if the *nice guy* is supportive of others, he should be able to count on the same level of support in return.

- The "I'll be there for you when you need me" contract: This contract is based on the belief that if the *nice guy* is available and helpful when others are in need, he should be able to rely on the same level of availability and help when he needs it.

- The "I'll do what you want if you do what I want" contract: This contract involves the idea that if the *nice guy* agrees to do what others want, he should be able to expect the same level of compromise in return.

- The "I'll be loyal to you if you're loyal to me" contract: This contract is based on the belief that if the *nice guy* is faithful and loyal to others, he should be able to expect the same level of loyalty in return.

- The "I'll forgive you if you forgive me" contract: This contract involves the idea that if the *nice guy* is willing to forgive others for their mistakes, he should be able to expect the same level of forgiveness in return.

- The "I'll be patient with you if you're patient with me" contract: This contract involves the idea that if the *nice guy* is patient and understanding with others, he should be able to expect the same level of patience and understanding in return.

- The "I'll be kind to you if you're kind to me" contract: This contract is based on the belief that if the *nice guy* is kind and compassionate to others, he should be able to expect the same level of kindness in return.

The problem with covert contracts is that, well,

they are covert. Imagine trying to build a house on top of a foundation hidden underground. No matter how much effort you put into constructing the walls and roof, the foundation will eventually crumble because it needs to be visible and supported. Similarly, covert contracts are like hidden foundations in relationships. They may initially seem stable but, ultimately, they cannot support the weight of the relationship because they need to be openly acknowledged and addressed. *Relationships built on covert contracts are prone to collapse because they are not grounded in open communication and mutual understanding.*

The Single Nice Guy and the Friendzone

I thought I was in love,
But she put me in the friendzone.
Now I'm her wingman,

Helping her find someone to bone.

Before Ryan developed a crush on Sara, he had a crush on a girl at work for many years, who had no interest in seeing him as more than a friendly colleague. Ryan was disappointed, but he believed he could get her to change her mind if he did things for her. Ryan offered to help her with her work and run errands for her. He tried to be there for her whenever she needed support or assistance. He tried to be extra kind and accommodating, hoping that this would make the girl see him as more than just a friend.

Despite his efforts, his colleague's feelings toward Ryan did not change. In fact, she often found Ryan overbearing and difficult to be around. Ryan couldn't shake his feelings of disappointment and resentment. He began to feel that he was being taken for granted and became angry and bitter. He started to feel like no matter how hard he tried, he would never be good enough for the girl he liked.

There are many possible reasons why Ryan might have been "friendzoned" by the girl he liked. It is not uncommon for individuals who exhibit the *Nice Guy Syndrome* to be seen as lacking in assertiveness or confidence, which are attractive qualities in a man.

Ryan's efforts to be kind and helpful were rightly perceived as lacking in authenticity or genuine interest, as he was motivated by a desire to gain the girl's affection.

Ryan's lack of communication and honesty about his feelings contributed to the girl not seeing him in a romantic light. By not expressing his desires and boundaries openly and honestly, he came across as lacking in assertiveness and self-respect.

To cope with his feelings, Ryan turned to unhealthy coping mechanisms. He began drinking heavily and partying excessively, hoping to numb his emotions and distract himself from his disappointment. He also started lashing out at others, including the girl he liked, becoming angry and aggressive when things didn't go his way.

These coping mechanisms provided temporary relief but ultimately worsened Ryan's situation. His other relationships suffered, and he felt even more isolated and unhappy. It wasn't until he hit rock bottom that Ryan realized he needed to make a change.

The Friendzone Is a Lonely Place

Single nice guys may feel jealous of those in relationships for various reasons. They may think they are missing out on the companionship and intimacy that comes with a relationship. They may also feel that they are not attractive or desirable to others, leading to insecurity and low self-esteem. In addition, they may think they cannot find someone who truly understands or appreciates them, leading to feelings of loneliness or isolation. Finally, they may feel that they cannot experience the joys and pleasures of being in a committed, loving relationship.

Ah, the age-old tale of the "nice guy" and the friendzone. Poor Ryan. He tried to be a good friend to the girl he liked, but unfortunately, his efforts to win her affection didn't quite pan out. But, hey, at least he tried.

But seriously, we've all been there. You want to be someone's friend, but secretly you're hoping for something more. And when that person doesn't feel the same way, it can be a tough pill to swallow. But as Ryan learned the hard way, trying to be someone's friend in the hopes of getting something in return is a recipe for disaster. It's better to be genuine and honest about your feelings.

And let's not forget about those unhealthy coping mechanisms. We've all turned to some questionable methods to deal with our disappointment at one time or another. But as Ryan discovered, they often make things worse.

Why Do Nice Guys Get Friendzoned?

There are several reasons why individuals who exhibit the *Nice Guy Syndrome* may get "friendzoned" by others, particularly when it comes to romantic relationships.

- They are seen as lacking in assertiveness or confidence, which are attractive qualities in a man, but they are too focused on pleasing their partners or potential love interests.

- They are too eager to please or willing to sacrifice their own needs and desires, which is perceived as lacking boundaries or self-respect.

- They are often perceived as manipulative or controlling, as they try to use their kindness or helpfulness to get what they secretly desire, which is often sex. They are usually not genuine in their actions, as their kindness is in the hope of getting something back.

- They struggle to express their feelings or desires openly and honestly, which makes it challenging to connect with them.

It is common for individuals who exhibit the *Nice Guy Syndrome* to become resentful when their efforts to gain love, affection, or validation are not rewarded. This is because they may feel that they have put in a lot of effort and made sacrifices but have yet to receive the recognition or appreciation they deserve.

This resentment is fueled by a belief that they are

entitled to a particular treatment for their actions. It can also be driven by feelings of frustration or disappointment, as the "nice guys" may feel that their attempts to be kind and helpful have not been effective.

Ultimately, this resentment can lead to anger, bitterness, or passive-aggressive actions. It can also lead to isolation or loneliness, as the "nice guys" may feel that they are not being understood or appreciated by others.

The Married Nice Guy

Neil's marital problems started long before he discovered his wife was cheating. Neil was married to a woman who was often critical and demeaning toward him. She criticized him for his flaws and mistakes and frequently compared him unfavorably to other men.

Neil's marriage was also sexless, and his wife frequently flirted with other men in front of him. She would tell him that she was frustrated by his lack of assertiveness and that he wasn't manly enough for her. Despite this treatment, Neil tried to be understanding and patient with his wife. He hoped that if he just tried harder to be a good husband, she would eventually appreciate him and treat him with more kindness and respect.

But his wife seemed to take him for granted the more he tried. She continued to belittle and insult him and showed no sign of changing her behavior. Neil became frustrated and resentful, and he began to feel like he was trapped in an unhappy and unfulfilling relationship.

To cope with these feelings, Neil began using pornography to escape his shame and disappointment. This provided temporary relief, but it ultimately made Neil feel worse about himself and his situation. He became isolated and disconnected from others and struggled to find healthy ways to deal with his frustration.

Nice Guys Frustrate Their Wives

Some specific behaviors that may frustrate a wife in a "nice guy" husband include:

- A lack of assertiveness or decision-making skills: "Nice guys" struggle to assert their own needs and desires, which can lead to a feeling of being overshadowed or ignored while simultaneously frustrating the partner if she needs to be in charge all the time.

- An inability to communicate openly and honestly: "Nice guys" have difficulty expressing their thoughts and feelings openly and honestly, which makes them come across as dishonest and secretive, leading to misunderstandings and conflicts.

- A tendency to be overly accommodating or self-sacrificial: "Nice guys" are often too eager to please or sacrifice their own needs and desires in an effort to be liked or approved of, which can be perceived as lacking in boundaries or self-respect.

- A tendency to be overly sensitive or reactive to criticism: "Nice guys" struggle to handle criticism or rejection and tend to become extremely sensitive or reactive when faced with these challenges.

- A lack of leadership or initiative: "Nice guys" struggle to take charge or make decisions, which leads to a feeling of being stuck or directionless.

- An inability to set boundaries: "Nice guys" have difficulty saying "no" or setting limits, which leads to feeling overwhelmed or taken advantage of.

- A lack of passion or ambition: "Nice guys" struggle to pursue their own goals or interests, which leads to a feeling of stagnation or lack of fulfillment.

The Nice Guy in the Workplace

"Nice Guys don't finish last; they rot in middle management." – Dr. Robert Glover

Nice Guy traits are not confined to dating or relationships. The Nice Guys' covert contracts often spill out into all areas and relationships of their lives, including friendships and at work.

Here are ways in which the *Nice Guy Syndrome* may manifest for men at work:

- A lack of assertiveness or confidence: "Nice guys" struggle to speak up for themselves or advocate for their own needs and ideas, limiting their professional advancement. Rowan was always hesitant to voice his opinions or to request a promotion or raise, even if he was qualified and deserving.

- An excessive focus on pleasing others or being liked: "Nice guys" prioritize being liked or approved of over their own needs or goals, which can lead to a lack of authenticity or genuine connection with colleagues. Rowan often agreed to take on additional tasks or responsibilities, even if it meant sacrificing his own time or well-being, to be appreciated.

- A lack of ambition or drive: "Nice guys" struggle to set and pursue their own goals, limiting their success and career advancement. Their drive is consumed by trying to please others, and they are often left with little energy to pursue their ambitions.

- An inability to handle criticism or feedback: "Nice guys" struggle to take constructive feedback or criticism, limiting their ability to learn and grow in their careers. Rowan would become defensive or upset when given feedback rather than viewing it as an opportunity for growth.

- A tendency to be overly accommodating or self-sacrificial: "Nice guys" are too eager to please or may sacrifice their own needs and desires in an effort to be liked or approved of, which can be seen as lacking in boundaries or self-respect. Rowan would consistently stay late or work weekends to help out a colleague, even if it meant sacrificing his own time or well-being.

- An inability to set boundaries: "Nice guys" have difficulty saying "no" or setting limits, which can lead to feeling overwhelmed or taken advantage of. Rowan consistently agreed to take on additional tasks to please others while deprioritizing his own assigned job responsibilities.

- A lack of leadership or initiative: "Nice guys" struggle to take charge or make decisions, which can lead to a lack of progress or direction in their work. Rowan was often hesitant to take on a leadership role or to initiate new projects or ideas for fear of failing, instead of seeing a new role as an opportunity to learn and grow.

- A tendency to be overly reactive or emotional: "Nice guys" struggle to manage their emotions or handle stress or challenges in a healthy way, affecting their performance and relationships with colleagues.

- An inability to handle conflict or confrontation: "Nice guys" struggle to address or resolve conflicts healthily and productively, which can lead to ongoing tensions or problems in the workplace.

- A lack of self-awareness: "Nice guys" are so outwardly focused on others' opinions that they struggle to recognize and understand their strengths and limitations, limiting their ability to grow and develop in their careers.

What Causes the Nice Guy Syndrome

Abandonment Anxiety and Toxic Shame

The fundamental causes of the *Nice Guy Syndrome* are the deadly one-two-punch combination of abandonment anxiety and toxic shame. Abandonment anxiety refers to a fear of being alone or rejected, which may stem from past experiences of neglect or rejection.

Toxic shame is an intense feeling of worthlessness and inadequacy often caused by adverse or traumatic experiences. It can be the result of abuse, neglect, or other forms of mistreatment, and it can profoundly impact the individuals' sense of self and their relationships with others. Toxic shame can lead to self-hatred, isolation, and a belief that one is fundamentally flawed or unworthy of love and acceptance. It can also cause people to engage in self-destructive behaviors or to become trapped in unhealthy or abusive relationships.

Neil was terrified of confronting his wife about her rude behavior and infidelity because he deeply feared being alone. This fear of abandonment stemmed from his childhood when he experienced a lot of instability and inconsistency in his family life. His parents divorced when he was young, and he often felt like he was being pushed to the side in favor of his siblings.

As an adult, Neil's abandonment anxiety manifested as a fear of being alone. He was always seeking out relationships and friendships, trying to fill the void of loneliness that he felt deep down. This led Neil to be a pushover in his marriage, going out of his way to avoid confrontation, even in the face of his wife's infidelity.

But Neil's nice guy tendencies didn't just manifest in his relationships. They also showed up in his work life, like with Rowan. Neil was often the first to volunteer for extra projects or tasks, even if it meant working long hours or sacrificing his own time and energy. He was terrified of being passed over for promotions or opportunities, so he'd do whatever it took to make himself indispensable to his boss and colleagues.

Unfortunately, Neil's need to please others and avoid rejection frequently backfired. Others often took advantage of him, and he would feel resentful and bitter when his efforts went unnoticed or unappreciated. His rejection sensitivity had also made it hard for him to be assertive in his relationships and set boundaries. He was afraid of being seen as "difficult" or "unlikeable," so he often tolerated behavior from others that he was not okay with.

Consequently, Neil's abandonment anxiety and rejection sensitivity caused him a lot of shame. He felt something was wrong with him for needing so much validation and attention from others. He often compared himself to others, feeling as if he was not good enough or worthy of love.

All of these issues contributed to Neil's *Nice Guy Syndrome*, and it was a constant struggle for him to break free from this pattern of behavior.

To cope with these feelings, Ryan, Neil, and Rowan turned to unhealthy self-soothing strategies like pornography, marijuana, and binge-watching YouTube videos. These activities provided temporary relief but ultimately left them feeling more disconnected and unfulfilled.

Abandonment anxiety and toxic shame can drive individuals to engage in behaviors that they believe will help them avoid being abandoned or rejected. In trying to be overly helpful or accommodating to win the approval or affection of others, *Nice Guys* avoid expressing their own needs or opinions in order to keep the peace. This leads to a cycle of seeking support and avoiding rejection, which can be emotionally and mentally draining.

It is vital for individuals with abandonment anxiety to recognize and address these underlying fears and to develop healthier ways of coping with their feelings.

- Rowan tried to be helpful and accommodating to his colleagues, even if it meant sacrificing his own needs and desires. He had a deep fear of being seen in a bad light, and he believed that if he were always there to help his colleagues and boss, they would like and accept him. However, these behaviors went unappreciated, and he frequently felt taken advantage of and resentful. He experienced shame over his own needs and desires and believed he was not worthy of having them met. He avoided expressing his own opinions or needs so as to appear to be low maintenance. He had a deep fear of being judged or rejected, and he believed that if he avoided rocking the boat, others would accept and like him. However, his lack of authenticity and honesty led to misunderstandings and conflicts, and he frequently felt resentful and unfulfilled.

- Neil avoided confrontation and difficult conversations with his wife to keep the peace. He had a deep fear of his wife leaving him, and he believed that if he avoided the hard conversations, his wife would change her ways. However, his avoidance often led to unresolved issues and ongoing tensions, and he frequently felt frustrated and resentful. He experienced shame over his own needs and boundaries, believing they were invalid or worthy of respect.

- Ryan constantly sought the approval and validation of the girls he liked. He had a deep fear of being rejected or disliked, and he believed that if he could prove himself to be "good enough," they would accept and like him. He frequently went out of his way to be helpful and avoided expressing what he truly wanted from them. However, despite his efforts, he felt inadequate and unfulfilled. Despite his shame, he continued to seek the approval of women to feel accepted and liked.

Rejection Sensitivity

Abandonment anxiety and shame contribute to the development of rejection sensitivity, which refers to a heightened sensitivity to being rejected or excluded. Individuals with high abandonment anxiety or guilt are prone to feeling rejected or excluded, even when that is not the case.

Rejection sensitivity eventually leads to the development of the *Nice Guy Syndrome*. To avoid being rejected or excluded, *Nice Guys* may engage in behaviors such as being overly helpful or accommodating or avoiding expressing their own needs or opinions. These behaviors are motivated by a desire for approval or acceptance, but they often have the opposite effect, as they lack authenticity and genuine interest. This creates a cycle of seeking approval and avoiding rejection, which drains precious life energy.

For example, an individual with abandonment anxiety may perceive a colleague's lack of response to their email as a sign of rejection, even if the colleague was busy or distracted. Similarly, an individual with shame may perceive minor criticism as evidence of their worthlessness or flaws rather than as an opportunity for growth or improvement.

Rowan has abandonment anxiety, manifesting as rejection sensitivity, and frequently interprets the actions of his colleagues as signs of rejection or disinterest. He becomes easily offended or hurt if someone doesn't respond to his email or if they don't include him in a group conversation, and he struggles to form genuine connections with others. His fear of being abandoned or rejected often leads him to avoid social situations or to seek constant reassurance from others, which in turn is draining for those around him. He takes even minor feedback or suggestions as evidence of his worthlessness or flaws, and he becomes easily defensive or upset when faced with criticism. As a result, he struggles to learn and grow in his career, and he often avoids taking on new challenges or risks out of fear of being rejected or judged.

Going Forward

In the remainder of this book, we will continue to follow Ryan, Neil, and Rowan as they take their *Hero's Journey* to *Nice Guy* recovery. Through their journeys, we will discover reliable and proven tools and strategies on the road to *integration*.

Getting Over the Nice Guy Syndrome

Three Conscious Decisions

When Nice Guys arrive at my doorstep (or Zoom room) for coaching, I ask them to commit to three decisions:

- A conscious decision to face fears
- A conscious decision to not settle for anything less than excellence
- A decision to make their own rules

This is also what I ask you to commit to as you continue on with the tools and strategies laid out in the rest of this book.

Yes, to stop being fraudulently nice is scary. But all recovering nice guys soon realize that most of their fears are irrational. Here are the five truths about fear as laid out brilliantly by Susan Jeffers Ph. D in her book *Feel The Fear And Do It Anyway®*.

FEAR TRUTH #1

The fear will never go away even as you continue to grow!

Every time you take a step into the unknown, you experience fear. There is no point in saying, "When I am no longer afraid, then I will do it." You'll be waiting for a long time. Fear is part of the package.

FEAR TRUTH #2

The only way to get rid of the fear of doing something is to go out and... do it!

Once you do it often enough, you will no longer be afraid in that particular situation. You will have faced the unknown, and you will have handled it. Then new challenges await you, which certainly add to the excitement of living.

FEAR TRUTH #3

The only way to feel better about yourself is to go out and... do it!

With each little step you take into unknown territory, a pattern of strength develops. You begin feeling stronger and stronger and stronger.

FEAR TRUTH #4

Not only are you afraid when facing the unknown, but so is everyone else!

This should be a relief. You are not the only one out there facing fear. Everyone feels fear when taking a step into the unknown. Yes, all those people who have succeeded in doing what they wanted to do have felt the fear – and did it anyway. So can you!

FEAR TRUTH #5

Pushing through fear is less frightening than living with the bigger underlying fear that comes from a feeling of helplessness!

This is the one truth that some people have difficulty understanding. When you push through the fear, you will feel such a sense of relief as your feeling of helplessness subsides. You will wonder why you did not take action sooner. You will become more and more aware that you can truly handle anything that life hands you.

Don't Do It Alone

Nice Guys are petrified of asking for help and feel incredibly uncomfortable when others try to give them help. They need to learn how to delegate tasks to others. Because they believe they have to do everything themselves, they rarely reach their full potential. And let's face it, nobody can be good at everything or succeed independently.

Breaking free from the *Nice Guy Syndrome* is no easy feat. It requires vulnerability and willingness to reveal oneself to safe individuals who can support them.

Make no mistake; finding a support system is non-negotiable. If you're serious about shedding the *nice guy persona* and becoming *you* unapologetically, you must seek out and surround yourself with safe individuals who can guide you on this journey.

So, for all the men ready to break free from the shackles of the *Nice Guy Syndrome*, hear me loud and clear: finding safe people to assist you in this process is essential. Not optional. You will not be able to do this on your own. It's time to reach out and create a support system. Your growth and development depend on it. Find a coach/therapist/men's group/safe group of friends willing to support you in your journey. Reach out to me at wildmancoaching.com for coaching or men's groups.

Who Is an Integrated Man?

Dr. Glover defines The Integrated Man is a man who has a healthy sense of self, who can balance the various aspects of his life, and who is comfortable in his own skin. He is aware of his own strengths and weaknesses. He tends to be authentic and honest and can express his thoughts and feelings healthily and appropriately. He no longer seeks external validation and acceptance from others but instead finds it from within. He can set healthy boundaries, assert himself, and communicate effectively, while being kind and compassionate. An integrated man understands that there are times when being assertive is necessary and when it is more appropriate to be more flexible. He can balance being strong and vulnerable. He takes responsibility for his happiness and does not depend on others to fulfill his emotional needs. He lives in alignment with his values and purpose.

The four traits of an integrated man according to Dr. Glover are:

- Self-soothing: He can soothe his anxiety in healthy ways to take action even when anxious.

- Conscious: He can be an observer of himself without judgment. Consciousness allows him to be present without ruminating about the past or fantasizing about the future.

- Differentiated: He can ask himself what he wants and what feels right and then hold on to that, despite pressure from others or his own anxiety and fear. He is comfortable being different from those around him in world view, values, ambitions, and preferences.

- Non-attached to Outcome: He is focused on the process of his choosing, on one that aligns with his values and purpose, and is not attached to what outcome it will produce. He is open to learning and growing, and adjusting along the way.

Learn to Self-Soothe

Self-soothing refers to the ability to calm oneself in the face of negative emotions or stress. It is an essential skill for anyone, especially nice guys, as it can help them manage their feelings and cope with difficult situations healthily and effectively.

The first step in Ryan's Nice Guy recovery journey was when he consciously tried to change his coping mechanisms – weed, porn, and YouTube. He started going to the gym regularly – lifting weights, running on the treadmill, and doing high-intensity interval training. He also started doing long hikes in nature and practicing yoga and meditation.

Through these strenuous exercises and mindfulness practices, he was able to calm his nervous system and reduce his anxiety. This made him feel and appear confident, and he built resistance against irrational sensitivity to rejection. He found that he could think more clearly, make better decisions, and feel more confident in his abilities.

Ryan's transformation didn't happen overnight, but with persistence and dedication, he could break free from the cycle of unhealthy self-soothing and reclaim his personal power.

The Nice Guy Syndrome can significantly impact an individual's nervous system, as the constant need to seek approval and avoid rejection can be emotionally and mentally draining. This can lead to an overactive stress response, adversely affecting physical and emotional well-being.

Chronic stress from constantly hiding and appearing needless can lead to various physical symptoms such as fatigue, difficulty sleeping, muscle tension, headaches, and digestive problems. It can also lead to emotional symptoms, such as irritability, difficulty concentrating, and feeling overwhelmed.

In addition, the constant effort to suppress one's needs and desires to be liked or accepted can lead to resentment and frustration, further contributing to stress and negative emotions.

Nice guys must recognize and address these behavior patterns and develop healthier ways of coping with stress and negative emotions.

Self-soothing can be especially important for nice guys who may have difficulty expressing their needs or setting boundaries. It can help them better manage their overwhelm or frustration and feel more in control of their lives.

Here's the thing: We will always find ways to soothe ourselves, but if we don't do it consciously, we will resort to unconscious and unhealthy patterns.

Some harmful or unhealthy ways that men try to self-soothe include:

- Using substances such as alcohol or drugs to numb or escape from negative emotions
- Engaging in risky or dangerous behaviors to distract themselves from anxiety
- Using food, porn, or other unhealthy habits
- Engaging in unhealthy relationships or behaviors as a way to find temporary relief
- Compulsively checking social media
- Using shopping or other forms of consumerism
- Engaging in self-harm
- Engaging in unhealthy or codependent relationships
- Using gambling or other forms of risky behavior as distractions

Strategies for Self-Soothing

Breathwork

"Breathing is the greatest pleasure in life."
– Giovanni Boccaccio

Breathwork is a simple and powerful self-soothing strategy for nice guys. It helps to calm the nervous system and promote relaxation in the face of negative emotions or stress.

Breathwork involves focusing on the breath to relax and manage stress. The breath is closely connected to our emotional and physical well-being, and by paying attention to and controlling the breath, we can have a positive impact on our overall health and well-being.

There are many different types of breathwork practices, and they all involve paying close attention to the breath and using specific breathing techniques to promote relaxation and stress management. Here are some easy and straightforward breathwork practices that can profoundly impact one's well-being.

Box Breathing

Box breathing is also known as square breathing or four-square breathing.

To practice box breathing, start by exhaling fully, then inhaling for a count of four. Hold your breath for a count of four, then exhale for a count of four. Hold your breath for a count of four, and then repeat the cycle.

One of the main advantages of box breathing is that it helps to slow down the breath and calm the nervous system, which can be beneficial for managing stress and anxiety. It is a simple and effective way to focus the mind and promote relaxation.

In addition, because it is a structured and repetitive practice, it's a valuable tool for developing mindfulness and focus. It can help individuals to tune out distractions and to stay present in the moment.

Box breathing is a simple practice that can be done anywhere and at any time, making it a convenient and effective self-soothing strategy for "nice guys."

4-7-8 Breathing

To practice 4-7-8 breathing, you start by exhaling fully through your mouth. Then, close your mouth and inhale quietly through your nose to a mental count of four. Hold your breath for a count of seven. Exhale completely through your mouth to a count of eight. This completes one breath. Now inhale again, and repeat the cycle for four breaths. That's it! This deceptively simple practice can profoundly lower stress levels and improve sleep. Because it involves a longer exhale than inhale, 4-7-8 breathing can help to activate the body's natural relaxation response.

Some other breathing techniques are:

Slow, deep breathing: This involves taking long, slow breaths in and out, focusing on the sensation of the breath moving in and out of the body.

Alternate nostril breathing: This involves closing one nostril and breathing in through the other nostril, then closing that nostril and exhaling through the opposite nostril. This can help to balance the nervous system and promote relaxation.

Belly breathing: This involves focusing on the movement of the belly by utilizing the diaphragm as you breathe in and out rather than the chest muscles. This can help to calm the nervous system and promote relaxation.

There are many free apps available that offer guided breathwork practices. Some popular options include:

- Headspace: This app offers a variety of meditation and mindfulness exercises, including breathwork practices. It is available for both iOS and Android.

- Calm: This app offers a range of mindfulness and relaxation exercises, including breathwork practices and guided meditations. It is available for both iOS and Android.

- Breathe: This app, available for iOS, offers a variety of breathing exercises and relaxation techniques. It includes a feature called "Breathe Reminders" that sends notifications to take a few minutes to breathe and relax throughout the day.

- Insight Timer: This app offers a wide range of meditation and mindfulness exercises, including breathwork practices and guided meditations. It is available for both iOS and Android.

Many other apps offer breathwork and relaxation exercises, so try a few different ones to find the one that works best.

Nature

"Nature's touch is gentle and kind –
A balm that soothes the troubled mind."

Spending time in nature can be a powerful self-soothing strategy. Nature has a calming and restorative effect on the mind and body and can help to shift the focus away from daily stressors and provide a sense of perspective and calm. Spending time in nature reliably improves mood, increases feelings of well-being, and reduces symptoms of depression. It can also improve cognitive function, creativity, and problem-solving skills.

Spending time in nature can be as simple as walking in a local park, hiking in the woods, or even just spending time in a backyard garden. Finding time to connect with nature regularly is essential, as the benefits can be long-lasting and profound.

Spending time in nature can be especially beneficial for nice guys as it can provide a sense of relaxation and calm in the face of negative emotions.

Strenuous Exercise

Strenuous exercise can be a way to self-soothe in several ways.

First, exercise releases endorphins which act as natural painkillers and mood elevators. In addition, exercise is a great way to shift the focus away from negative thoughts or emotions and to channel energy into something positive and productive. The physical and mental challenges of strenuous exercise provide a sense of accomplishment and self-esteem.

For the nice guy, exercise can provide a healthy outlet for this built-up tension. In addition, nice guys may struggle with low self-esteem and benefit from the sense of accomplishment and self-esteem that comes from strenuous exercise. This can help to improve overall confidence and self-worth.

Finally, exercise can provide a chance to connect with others and to find social support, which can be especially helpful for nice guys who may struggle with feelings of isolation or loneliness.

Exercise can provide a sense of community and a chance to connect with others with similar interests and goals.

Here are five fun ways to get strenuous exercises regularly:

- Rock climbing: Rock climbing is a physically and mentally challenging exercise that requires strength, endurance, and problem-solving skills. It can be done indoors or outdoors and can be a great way to challenge yourself and improve overall fitness.

- High-intensity interval training (HIIT): HIIT is a type of exercise involving short bursts of intense activity followed by brief rest periods. It can be done with various movements, including running, cycling, or strength training, and is a great way to improve cardiovascular fitness and build muscle.

- Kickboxing: Kickboxing is a high-intensity

cardiovascular exercise combining boxing and martial arts elements. It is a great way to improve coordination, balance, and flexibility and can be a fun and challenging way to get a full-body workout.

- CrossFit: CrossFit is a high-intensity strength and conditioning program combining weightlifting, gymnastics, and cardiovascular exercise elements. It is a great way to improve overall fitness and can be a fun and challenging way to get in shape.

- Surfing: Surfing is a physically and mentally challenging sport that requires strength, endurance, and balance. It is a great way to improve overall fitness and can be a fun and exciting way to enjoy the outdoors.

Rowan takes his First Step in his Nice Guy Recovery

Rowan had always been self-conscious about his

body and struggled with anxiety for as long as he could remember. He knew that he needed to make a change, but he didn't know where to start. That's when he stumbled upon a CrossFit box (a bare-bones gym) near his home.

He had heard about CrossFit before but was slightly intimidated by the idea of working out with strangers. But he decided to take the plunge and join the box. He was surprised at how welcoming the community was and how quickly he made friends. He felt a sense of camaraderie and support among the members he had never experienced.

The workouts were challenging, but he found that he was capable of more than he had ever thought possible. He was amazed at how quickly he could see improvements in his strength, endurance, and flexibility. He was proud of his progress, which helped him feel more confident and less anxious.

As Rowan continued to train, he began to notice that he was getting some attention from girls. His newfound confidence, strength, and discipline positively impacted his overall energy.

Meditation

Let's cut to the chase. Mindfulness meditation is no longer just for hippies and Zen monks. It's a powerful tool that more and more people are turning to for managing stress, boosting performance, and improving overall well-being.

In recent years, there's been an explosion of interest in mindfulness. And for good reason. The research is clear: mindfulness can reduce symptoms of anxiety and depression, improve attention and focus, and increase emotional regulation. It's not just some woo-woo mumbo jumbo; it's science.

But it's not just researchers who are taking notice. Businesses, healthcare organizations, and educational institutions are incorporating mindfulness practices to boost performance and well-being. The growing awareness and acceptance of mindfulness in mainstream society have made it more accessible than ever.

We all need tools to manage the mind, and mindfulness is one of the most accessible, effective, and efficient tools out there. So, it's time to embrace mindfulness for those looking to level up and take charge of their mental and emotional well-being. Trust me, you won't regret it.

There are many different types of meditation, including:

- Mindfulness meditation: This type of meditation involves focusing on the present moment and bringing awareness to one's thoughts, feelings, and sensations without judgment.

- Loving-kindness meditation: This type of meditation involves silently repeating phrases of love and compassion to oneself and others.

- Transcendental meditation: This type of meditation involves silently repeating a mantra or phrase to oneself to quiet the mind and achieve a state of relaxation.

- Guided meditation: This type of meditation involves following the guidance of a recorded voice or live instructor to help bring focus and relaxation to mind.

- Yoga meditation: This type of meditation combines physical poses with breathing techniques and focused attention to bring relaxation and clarity to mind.

Meditation is essential for nice guys as it can help improve self-awareness and self-regulation and provide a healthy outlet for managing stress and negative emotions.

Here are a few free apps that can be used to practice meditation:

- Headspace: Headspace is a popular meditation app that offers guided meditation and mindfulness exercises for beginners and experienced meditators alike. It has many topics, including stress, sleep, and focus.
- Calm: Calm is another popular app that offers guided meditation and mindfulness exercises, sleep stories, breathing exercises, and relaxation music.
- Insight Timer: Insight Timer is a meditation app that offers a variety of guided meditations and mindfulness exercises, as well as a library of over 60,000 music tracks and talks. It also has a social component, allowing users to connect with other meditators and join virtual

meditation groups.

- The Mindfulness App: The Mindfulness App is a meditation app that offers guided meditation and mindfulness exercises, as well as a timer for silent reflection. It also has a feature that allows users to set reminders to practice mindfulness throughout the day.

- Omvana: Omvana is a meditation app that offers a variety of guided meditations and mindfulness exercises, as well as a library of over 500 tracks for relaxation and sleep. It also has a feature that allows users to create their own meditation playlists.

Vipassana: Ten Days that Can Change Your Life

Are you ready to elevate your mind and body to new heights? Look no further than Vipassana meditation. This little-known practice has been a not-so-secret weapon in my nice guy recovery journey for the past 12 years.

I attended my first ten-day silent Vipassana retreat 12 years ago, and it was a complete game-changer. Not only did I feel calmer, less reactive to stress, and more focused, but I also experienced physical health benefits like reduced blood pressure and less chronic pain.

I have since made it a regular part of my routine. Every year, I attend a Vipassana retreat, and with each one, I feel younger, healthier, calmer, more productive, and more creative. It's like hitting the reset button on my mind and body.

And here's the best part: it's entirely free, based on the donation economy, so no one is turned away for lack of funds.

If you want to take your ability to self-soothe to a superhuman level, check out Vipassana, as taught by S.N. Goenka. Go to www.dhamma.org to find a ten-day retreat near you; trust me, you won't regret it.

Neil Makes a Decision to Prioritize His Needs

Neil was at a breaking point. I suggested he take a ten-day Vipassana retreat. At first, Neil was hesitant. He was scared of taking so much time away from his family and work. But I encouraged him to assert his needs, and to his surprise, his wife and boss readily agreed.

Neil decided to take the plunge and signed up for the retreat. It wasn't easy for him to take ten days away from everything and everyone he knew, but he knew it was necessary for his mental and emotional well-being.

During the retreat, Neil felt more peaceful and in control of his thoughts.

When he came back, he felt rejuvenated. He was

surprised that no one had objected to him taking time off and realized that all his fears were just in his own head. He was grateful to have taken the time for himself and knew he needed to continue doing it for his own well-being. He felt re-energized and grounded. The ten days spent in silence and solitude had allowed him to clear his mind and gain a new perspective on life. He felt more in tune with his needs and was now more assertive in communicating them to those around him.

He returned to his work and personal life with a renewed sense of purpose and was more productive and creative. He was determined to continue this practice and make it a regular routine.

Learn to be Conscious

Recovering from the Nice Guy Syndrome requires a conscious effort to understand and change long-standing patterns of behavior. Consciousness is the foundation of self-awareness, which is critical to overcoming the Nice Guy Syndrome.

Being conscious means being an observer of oneself without judgment. It allows one to be present without ruminating about the past or fantasizing about the future. It involves recognizing and accepting one's thoughts, feelings, and behaviors in the present moment, without trying to control or manipulate them.

Leading thinkers in this area, such as Eckhart Tolle and Jon Kabat-Zinn, recommend mindfulness meditation as a way to cultivate consciousness. This involves focusing attention on the present moment and observing thoughts and sensations without judgment. This practice can help one become more aware of automatic patterns of behavior and thought, and help to break those patterns.

Another strategy is to practice self-reflection, which involves regularly examining one's thoughts, feelings, and behaviors to gain insight into patterns and tendencies. Psychologists such as Carl Jung and Virginia Satir have emphasized the importance of self-reflection for personal growth and development. This can be done through journaling, therapy, or discussing with a trusted friend or mentor.

Moving forward, it's important to recognize that becoming more conscious is not a one-time event, but a lifelong journey. As you continue this journey, you will begin to see the world and yourself in new ways. You will start to see the patterns of your thoughts and behaviors, and you will be able to make conscious choices that align with your values.

In the next chapter, we'll discuss how to take that self-awareness and use it to prioritize yourself. We'll explore why prioritizing oneself is critical to breaking free from the Nice Guy Syndrome, and learn strategies for overcoming obstacles and guilt associated with putting oneself first. By prioritizing oneself, one can cultivate a sense of self-worth and create healthier relationships with others.

Learn to Prioritize Yourself

"The truth will set you free, but first it will piss you off." – Gloria Steinem

Do you get tired of feeling like the nice guy who never seems to get what he wants? There is a common flawed strategy that holds nice guys back: trying to become "needless and wantless."

Many of us, especially those who experienced childhood abandonment, believe that our needs and wants drive people away. We think that if we could just eliminate or hide those needs, we'd never be abandoned again. But here's the thing: it's impossible to completely repress our needs and still survive.

So what do we do? We try to appear like we don't

have any needs while trying to get them met indirectly and in covert ways. But this creates an unsolvable paradox: we can't totally repress our needs and stay alive, and we can't meet our needs on our own.

It's time to break this cycle and learn to assert your needs healthily and directly. Avoid falling for the trap of thinking that having few needs or wants is a virtue. The truth is we all have needs, and it's essential to learn how to meet them in a healthy way.

So, let's change the narrative, embrace your needs and wants, and learn to assert them in a healthy way. It's time to level up your life, and it all starts with understanding and accepting that you have needs and that it is okay to have them.

Everything a nice guy does is consciously or unconsciously calculated to gain someone's approval or avoid disapproval. And now we know the reason why – rejection sensitivity. So, a safe way to start working with increasing your resilience against rejection sensitivity is to rely on the one person you have the most control over – and that is YOU.

Before we identify our needs, it's essential to understand how we try to "fit in" in attempting to appear needless and wantless while covertly still trying to get our needs met.

Identify Your Approval-Seeking Behavior

Go through the list provided below and see which behaviors resonate with you. Some of these behaviors may be more subtle or unconscious, but taking the time to become aware of them is a necessary step in the recovery process. As you go through the list, consider how each behavior manifests in your daily life and how it may impact your relationships and overall well-being. Remember, the goal is not to shame or blame yourself but to gain insight and understanding to make positive changes.

- Covertly seeking validation from others or asking for constant reassurance from others
- Putting others' needs before your own
- Struggling to say "no" or set boundaries
- Struggling to express your opinions and needs to others
- Avoiding confrontation or disagreement
- Going along with others' plans even when you don't want to
- Avoiding expressing anger or frustration
- Being overly accommodating
- Being overly generous
- Seeking to be needed by others
- Avoiding speaking up in group settings
- Believing that one must be perfect to be loved or worthy

Identify Where You Are "Faking It"

It's time to take a hard look at yourself and see if you're guilty of any of these sneaky tactics to cover up your flaws. Are you constantly "faking it" by pretending to be someone you're not to impress others? Or are you resorting to "fixing" things for others to win their approval? It's essential to be honest with yourself about these behaviors. Don't hide behind these convenient masks – it's time to get real.

- Faking kindness, generosity
- Faking selflessness, humility
- Faking vulnerability
- Faking empathy or support
- Faking honesty
- Faking interest or agreement
- Faking respect or appreciation
- Faking affection
- Faking compliance or obedience

- Faking loyalty or commitment
- Pretending to be something you are not
- Hiding your true intentions, emotions, or reactions
- Lying or withholding information
- Faking achievements or successes
- Masking your flaws or weaknesses
- Faking compatibility or shared values or shared interests
- Faking a sense of shared history or connection
- Faking a sense of shared destiny or future together
- Faking a sense of shared identity or belonging
- Faking a sense of shared purpose or meaning
- Faking a sense of shared vision or goals
- Faking a sense of shared values or morals
- Faking a sense of shared spirituality or faith
- Faking a sense of shared cultural or social background

- Faking a sense of shared lifestyle or preferences
- Faking a sense of shared tastes or hobbies

Learn to Identify and Name Your Needs

Before you move any further, familiarize yourself with these universal human needs. Everything we humans do in life at any time is in service of trying to meet one or more of these needs. Being able to identify and name our needs for ourselves and others is the first step in getting those needs met. These needs are fundamental life-affirming resources that help us survive and thrive.

Acceptance, belonging, affection, air, appreciation, authenticity, clarity, cooperation, love, communication, closeness, food, play, community, companionship, touch, compassion, consideration, consistency, empathy, inclusion, integrity, intimacy, mutuality, nurturing, respect/self-respect, safety, security, shelter, stability, support, trust, warmth, water, movement, exercise, rest, sleep, sexual expression, play, joy, humor, peace, beauty, communion, ease, equality, harmony, inspiration, order, autonomy, choice, freedom, independence, space, spontaneity, celebration, challenge, competence, consciousness, contribution, creativity, discovery, effectiveness, growth, hope, learning, mourning, participation, purpose, self-expression, to matter, to know and be known, to see and be seen, to understand and be understood

And now, let's get to the actual work. For each of your covert, approval-seeking behaviors or the ways that you fake being "needless and wantless," it's time to take a closer look and start asserting your needs in a healthy and direct manner. This may require self-reflection and honesty about what you truly need, but it's crucial to leveling up your life and improving your relationships.

Identify your motivations: Why do you need to pretend or hide your true self? What needs are you trying to get met through all this faking? Refer to the lists above.

Practice honesty: Start small by being honest with yourself and those around you about your thoughts, feelings, and desires. This can be challenging at first, but it can also be liberating and empowering.

Seek support: Talk to a trusted friend, family member, or professional about your struggles with authenticity. Someone supporting you and holding you accountable can make a big difference.

Rowan Gets a Wake Up Call

Rowan would constantly try to please his boss at work. He also found himself frequently seeking the approval of his friends, always trying to be the life of the party and go along with whatever they wanted to do.

Deep down, Rowan knew this constant need for approval wasn't healthy. He felt like he was always putting on a show and never truly being himself. He started to feel drained and unfulfilled by these behaviors.

Rowan's boss called him into her office for a performance review one day. Rowan had always tried his best to be the perfect employee. But as he sat in her office, his boss informed him that while trying to be helpful around the office, he was behind in meeting his own goals. His attitude was actually hindering his growth and development within the company.

Rowan was taken aback by this feedback. This moment was a turning point for Rowan. He realized his constant need for approval damaged his career and personal relationships. He started working on himself, focusing on his goals and desires and practicing honesty and authenticity in all interactions. He decided that enough was enough. He began to dig deep and examine the motivations behind his need for approval. He realized that much of it stemmed from his insecurities and a fear of rejection. He knew he needed to make a change. He sought support from friends and a therapist to help him overcome his insecurities.

He started to speak up and express his opinions and priorities rather than just trying to please others. As he let go of these unhealthy approval-seeking behaviors, Rowan began to feel more authentic and true to himself. He found that he could form deeper, more fulfilling connections with others. He no longer needed to put on a show and could just be himself.

Start with the Basics

One of the most effective strategies is to create a weekly plan that incorporates a variety of self-care, personal growth, boundary-setting, and emotional well-being activities. My suggestion? Choose a few items from each category, and make them non-negotiable parts of your schedule. For instance, commit to exercising three times a week, spend time in nature on the weekends, and set aside daily moments for solitude or contemplation. Additionally, consider adding personal growth practices like working on a goal or taking up a creative hobby. By designing a weekly routine that includes these activities, you'll be able to cultivate a more fulfilling and well-rounded life.

Here are 40 practical things that "Nice Guys" can do for themselves to feel good:

Self-Care:

- Get enough sleep each night
- Exercise regularly
- Eat a healthy diet
- Take breaks to relax and recharge
- Engage in hobbies that bring joy
- Treat yourself to a massage or other spa services
- Take a day trip or weekend getaway
- Learn a new skill or hobby
- Practice relaxation techniques like deep breathing or meditation
- Get a new haircut or change your hairstyle
- Invest in new clothes or accessories that make you feel confident
- Take up a physical activity like dancing, yoga, or martial arts

Emotional Well-Being:

- Write down things you are grateful for and share your gratitude with others
- Appreciate the beauty around you
- Seek therapy or counseling or join a support group
- Spend time with supportive friends and family
- Go for a walk or spend time in nature
- Read a book or watch a movie for pleasure
- Take a relaxing bath
- Set aside time each day for solitude or quiet contemplation

Personal Growth and Development:

- Volunteer your time to a cause you care about
- Practice self-compassion and learn to speak kindly to yourself
- Set goals for yourself and work toward achieving them

- Practice forgiveness and let go of grudges
- Take up a creative outlet like painting, writing, or music
- Seek out positive role models or mentors
- Seek out opportunities for social connection and community
- Get outside your comfort zone and try something new and exciting

Setting Boundaries:

- Limit time with draining people
- Say "no" to unreasonable requests
- Set limits on availability

More on boundaries in a later chapter.

Neil Takes Responsibility for His Well-Being

As Neil approached his mid-thirties, he began to feel burned out and unfulfilled. He realized that he had been neglecting his own well-being for far too long.

He decided to focus on the basics of self-care. He started exercising regularly and eating a healthy, balanced diet. He also got plenty of rest, setting aside time each night to relax and unwind before bed.

He worked on improving his emotional well-being. He began practicing mindfulness and meditation, which he learned in a Vipassana retreat, which helped him to better manage his stress and emotions. He also started weekly coaching sessions with me, which provided him with a safe space to explore his feelings and learn new coping mechanisms.

Ryan Sets Healthy Boundaries

Slowly, Ryan learned the importance of setting boundaries. With the newfound vocabulary of his own needs, he communicated his needs and limits clearly to others. This helped him feel more in control of his life and relationships and allowed him to focus on his priorities. One of the biggest challenges Ryan faced was setting boundaries with his mother. He had always struggled to assert himself with her, but he knew it was essential for his well-being. So, he began practicing saying "no" and setting clear limits with her. It wasn't easy but, over time, Rowan learned to stand up for himself and set healthy boundaries with the people in his life.

Self-Approval

"What do I want?" "What feels right to me?" "What would make me happy?"

Make Your Own Rules

The recovering nice guy's number one priority has to be to move from seeking external validation to generating self-approval. Nice Guys spend all their lives trying to fit into others' definition of a good life at the cost of sacrificing their desires. Seldom do they realize that the privilege of being adults is that we get to make our own rules, live by them, and accept the consequences.

Toward the end of his book, Dr. Glover lays out 30 Rules for nice guys to try on for size. These rules are:

1. If it frightens you, do it.
2. Don't settle. Every time you settle, you get exactly what you settled for.
3. Put yourself first.
4. No matter what happens, you will handle it.
5. Whatever you do, do it 100%.
6. If you do what you have always done, you will get what you have always gotten.
7. You are the only person on this planet responsible for your needs, wants, and happiness.

8. Ask for what you want.

9. If what you are doing isn't working, try something different.

10. Be clear and direct.

11. Learn to say "no."

12. Don't make excuses.

13. If you are an adult, you are old enough to make your own rules.

14. Let people help you.

15. Be honest with yourself.

16. Do not let anyone treat you badly. No one. Ever.

17. Remove yourself from a bad situation instead of waiting for the situation to change.

18. Don't tolerate the intolerable – ever.

19. Stop blaming. Victims never succeed.

20. Live with integrity. Decide what feels right to you, then do it.

21. Accept the consequences of your actions.

22. Be good to yourself.

23. Think "abundance."

24. Face difficult situations and conflict head-on.

25. Don't do anything in secret.

26. Do it now.

27. Be willing to let go of what you have to get what you want.

28. Have fun. If you are not having fun, something is wrong.

29. Give yourself room to fail. There are no mistakes, only learning experiences.

30. Control is an illusion. Let go; let life happen.

Which of these rules do you already live by? Which of these rules are scary to you? Which of these rules are you willing to risk incorporating into your life?

My friend and colleague Chuck Chapman has written an excellent companion journal to help nice guys live into these rules. I encourage you to grab his book and work through incorporating these rules into your life. You can find the book at: https://amzn.to/4oAwDI3

Ryan Confronts His Insecurities

With my guidance, Ryan began focusing on self-care and well-being. He started exercising regularly, meditating daily, and taking up hobbies that he enjoyed. He also began to work on his emotional intelligence, learning how to express his feelings and set healthy boundaries with others.

As he prioritized his needs, Ryan began feeling more confident and self-assured. He stopped putting up with disrespectful or unhealthy behavior from his friends and started standing up for himself more.

Ryan also started to take risks and embrace new experiences. He started saying "yes" to invitations and opportunities that he would have previously turned down out of fear or insecurity. This led to some mistakes and learning experiences in the dating world, but he learned from them and moved on.

One of the most significant breakthroughs for Ryan came when he started a gratitude practice. He began to focus on all of the good things in his life rather than dwelling on his flaws and insecurities. This shift in perspective helped him acknowledge all of the abundance around him and move away from a scarcity mentality.

Rowan Moves Toward Self-Acceptance

Rowan had always been a perfectionist, and this tendency had often caused him to be overly critical of himself and others. He slowly learned to accept and embrace his quirks and flaws. This included his perfectionism, love for collecting rare stamps, and penchant for singing loudly in the shower. Rather than hiding these quirks or trying to change them, he learned to embrace them and even find humor in them. This newfound self-acceptance made him more interesting and endearing to others.

Learn to Differentiate Yourself

"Your time is limited, don't waste it living someone else's life."

- Steve Jobs

As a recovering Nice Guy, one of the biggest challenges you face is learning to differentiate yourself from others. This means being able to know yourself, your values, your beliefs, and your goals, and to express them without fear or shame. It requires the courage to make your own decisions, even if they go against the opinions of others.

Differentiation is the opposite of fusion, which is the tendency to merge with others and lose your own sense of self. When you are fused, you may find yourself sacrificing your own needs and desires for the sake of others, or being overly concerned with their opinions and feelings. This can lead to feelings of resentment and frustration.

To become differentiated, you must first identify your own needs and desires. This means asking yourself what you want and what feels right, without worrying about what others may think or say. It requires being honest with yourself and acknowledging your feelings, even if they are uncomfortable.

Once you have identified your own needs and desires, it's important to hold onto them, even when faced with pressure from others or your own anxiety and fear. This means being comfortable with being different from those around you, and standing up for what you believe in.

However, practicing differentiation can be challenging and may result in opposition from others who are used to you being a certain way. In these moments, it's important to practice self-soothing techniques to help you stay grounded and centered.

It's important to note that differentiation doesn't mean deliberately going against what someone is saying or doing. Rather, it's about conscious fusion instead of fusing for the sake of validation. It's about being able to take in what others are saying, consider their perspective, and then decide what is right for you.

Differentiation is a crucial step in building your masculine identity, which will be discussed in the next chapter. It's also an essential part of setting healthy boundaries, which will be explored in the chapter following that.

Remember, unconscious fusion is the enemy of differentiation. When you fuse with others, you lose your own sense of self and become dependent on their approval and validation. By practicing differentiation and self-soothing techniques, you can break free from this pattern and become the confident, self-assured person you were meant to be.

Build Your Masculine Identity

Why Do Nice Guys Tend to Distrust Other Men?

Nice Guys often distrust other men because they have been taught that traditional masculinity is toxic or undesirable. They usually grow up without positive male role models and have had negative experiences with men who embody traditional masculine traits such as aggression or competitiveness. As a result, Nice Guys often feel like they have to distance themselves from these traits to be accepted by others, particularly women. This can lead to mistrust and resentment toward other men who exhibit these traits.

The nice guy may feel jealous or threatened by a

male colleague who is confident and assertive in the workplace, even if that colleague is not necessarily trying to be aggressive or dominating. The nice guy may view the confident colleague as a threat to his own success or sense of worth. He may feel like he has to constantly prove himself to the confident colleague, leading to feelings of inadequacy and resentment.

Another example might be a Nice Guy who feels he has to hide his interests or hobbies to fit in with his female friends. It's not uncommon for men to suppress their love of sports or action movies to be considered sensitive or caring, leading to a disconnection from other men who share these interests.

Masculine energy is associated with strength, discipline, courage, passion, persistence, assertiveness, ambition, and integrity. It is often associated with traditional male roles and behaviors. These qualities and energies are not exclusive to one gender or another, and individuals of any gender can exhibit both masculine and feminine energies. However, because they mistrust men, nice guys often tend to be afraid or ashamed of the very masculine energies that empower a man to create and produce amazing things in the world. This masculine energy also empowers them to provide for and protect those important to them.

Connect with Emotionally Healthy Men

Connecting with men is essential for reclaiming masculinity. Building relationships with men requires a conscious effort, and this process begins with a commitment to developing male friendships. To do this, recovering nice guys must be willing to make the time, take risks, and be vulnerable. This can involve joining a team, attending sporting events, a prayer or discussion group, having a poker night, doing volunteer work, fishing, running, or just hanging out. It's essential to find activities that align with your interests and values and to be willing to try new things. By building strong, authentic relationships with men, you can gain a sense of camaraderie and belonging that is essential for a healthy sense of masculinity.

Get Strong

Enhancing physical strength can be a powerful tool in reclaiming masculinity for nice guys. Whether through weightlifting, martial arts, or other forms of exercise, building strength and endurance improves physical health and helps individuals feel more confident and capable. This process requires dedication, discipline, and a willingness to push oneself beyond comfort zones, all of which are essential aspects of masculinity. By embracing the challenge of becoming stronger, nice guys can tap into their inner power and assertiveness, reclaiming their masculinity and personal power.

Find Healthy Male Role Models

Finding mentors and role models who embody healthy masculinity can help nice guys reclaim their masculinity. By observing and learning from these individuals, we can gain insights and strategies for embodying masculinity in a healthy and authentic way. There are many places where we can seek out healthy male role models. Some options include seeking out mentors or coaches within the professional field, joining a men's group or fraternity, participating in activities or organizations that align with your values and interests, or simply seeking out friends and peers who embody the qualities and characteristics you admire. We must be proactive and intentional in our search for role models, as these individuals can provide valuable guidance, support, and accountability.

The Father Wound

The distrust in men can also often be traced back to The Father Wound. The Father Wound describes the emotional pain and trauma resulting from a man's relationship with his father. This wound can manifest in various ways, including inadequacy, anger, and a lack of purpose or direction in life. It can also manifest as a profound disconnection from others and difficulty forming and maintaining close relationships.

It is crucial to approach the topic of the father wound with compassion and understanding to create a safe and supportive space for healing.

Working with a therapist or counselor can be a

helpful way to explore and process the emotions and experiences associated with the "Father Wound." A therapist can provide a safe and supportive space to process and heal from the pain of the past. Having emotionally healthy men in your life can be incredibly helpful in the healing process. These men can serve as role models and mentors, helping to provide guidance, support, and a sense of connection.

Examining their relationship with their fathers helps Nice Guys see them as they are rather than idealizing or demonizing them. This may involve anger or rage, even if their fathers are no longer alive. The important thing is to embrace the shared male heritage and view fathers as flawed but still worthy human beings. This shift allows Nice Guys to better understand and accept themselves and reclaim their masculinity.

Healing from the "Father Wound" is a journey that will likely involve ups and downs. It is essential to be patient with oneself and seek support and resources to help on this journey. Healing and finding greater peace are possible with time, patience, and the right resources.

Summary

Building a masculine identity is about being unapologetically yourself. It's not about conforming to societal expectations or hiding behind a facade of perfection. It's about embracing our flaws, owning our imperfections, and occupying our place in the world with confidence and ownership.

It's time to break free from the notion that men must be strong, unbreakable, and always in control. The truth is we all have moments of doubt and insecurity. And that's okay. Embracing our vulnerabilities is not a sign of weakness but strength. It takes courage to be open and honest about our struggles and insecurities; but through this openness, we can connect with others and build meaningful relationships.

As men, it's crucial to take ownership of our actions. This means being responsible for our choices and standing up for our beliefs. It's about being accountable for our actions and taking responsibility for our impact on us and others.

Building a masculine identity is recognizing that we are worthy and deserving of love, respect, and acceptance. It's about understanding that our unique strengths and abilities are valuable and that we have a role to play in this world.

Set Healthy Boundaries

Here is something I tell my clients, which they often find triggering and makes them want to punch me: "If someone continues to treat you badly, it's your fault. To stop tolerating someone's bad behavior is not just completely in your control – it's your responsibility to yourself."

Boundaries are the limits we set for ourselves regarding what we are willing to tolerate, accept, or do in a relationship. They help us protect our physical, emotional, and mental well-being and establish a sense of respect and autonomy in our relationships.

Boundaries can be physical, such as setting limits around personal space or touch, or emotional, such as how others can speak to us or what we are willing to share about ourselves. Boundaries can also be behavioral, such as setting limits around what we are willing to do or not do in a relationship.

In healthy relationships, both parties respect each other's boundaries and work to establish a sense of mutual respect and understanding. Setting and maintaining boundaries is essential to self-care and can help individuals cultivate healthy, fulfilling relationships.

Why Do Nice Guys Struggle with Setting Boundaries?

Nice guys struggle with boundaries for a variety of reasons. Some common underlying causes include:

1. A lack of awareness of their own needs: Nice Guys may have difficulty setting boundaries

because they are not fully aware of their own needs and values. With a strong self-awareness, it can be easier to identify what is and is not acceptable to them in any relationship.

2. A fear of confrontation or rejection: Nice guys have difficulty setting boundaries because they fear conflict or rejection. They often prioritize maintaining harmony in their relationships over standing up for themselves or setting limits with others.

3. A tendency to put others' needs ahead of their own: Nice guys struggle with boundaries because they tend to put others' needs ahead of their own. They may prioritize pleasing others or avoiding conflict over standing up for themselves and expressing their needs and wants.

Early relationships with parents can play a significant role in developing people-pleasing tendencies and a person's ability to set and maintain boundaries.

If a Nice Guy grew up in a household where their parents did not set clear boundaries or did not respect their boundaries, they might not have learned how to set boundaries themselves. For example, suppose a child's parents regularly intrude on their privacy or make decisions without considering their thoughts or feelings. In that case, they may not have learned how to assert their boundaries. People-pleasing tendencies can often be related to early relationships with parents, mainly if a child's needs are not consistently met or their boundaries are not respected. When parents are always critical or demanding, children can develop a strong desire to please their parents to avoid criticism or rejection.

On the other hand, a child who grows up in a

house where the parents are consistently nurturing and responsive to their needs may be more likely to develop a strong sense of self-worth and assertiveness.

Identifying Your Values and Limits

The first step in asserting your boundaries is identifying your values and limits. We need to know our boundaries to expect others to know them. Let's get to work.

Reflect on past experiences: Take time to think about past experiences in relationships and how they have shaped your beliefs and behaviors. Consider any patterns or themes that emerge, such as when you felt unsupported or put others' needs ahead of your own or when what others did or said upset you. All these triggers provide clues to your acceptable behavior limit or boundaries.

Identify your non-negotiables: Make a list of the things that are most important to you and that you are not willing to compromise on in a relationship. These include respect, honesty, or physical touch.

Seek feedback from trusted friends and loved ones: Ask them for their input on your values and limits. They can provide valuable insight and perspective on your beliefs and behaviors.

Practice setting boundaries: Start small by setting boundaries in small, low-risk situations. For example, you might practice saying "no" when someone asks you to do something you don't want to do. As you become more comfortable setting boundaries, you can start setting them in more significant situations.

Seek support from a therapist or counselor: Working with a trained professional can be a helpful way to explore your values and limits and develop strategies for setting and maintaining healthy boundaries in your relationships.

By engaging in these activities, the nice guy can understand his values and limits and establish healthy boundaries in his relationships.

Communicating Boundaries Assertively

Dr. Glover says, "We must train people how we want them to treat us. A strong, healthy man shows his partner (or people in his life) how he expects her to be in their relationship and then leads her into that place with love and integrity. It's not about control, and it certainly isn't about waiting for her to figure it out on her own."

Here are some ways to communicate assertively:

- Use "I" statements: Instead of making accusations or placing blame, use "I" statements to express your feelings and experiences. For example, instead of saying, "You're always late," try saying, "I feel disrespected when you are consistently late for our plans. I would like you to start coming to our planned meeting on time."

- Be specific: Clearly and specifically articulate your boundaries and what you are and are not willing to tolerate. Avoid vague or ambiguous language.

- Be firm but respectful: Be firm in expressing your boundaries, but do so respectfully. Avoid aggression or sarcasm.

- Practice assertiveness: Assertiveness is a skill that can be developed with practice. Start by setting boundaries in small, low-risk situations and gradually work your way up to more significant boundaries.

- Be willing to walk away, temporarily or permanently: If you aren't ready to walk away from an intolerable or unsatisfactory situation, you have no power to change the situation. Everyone involved will know it. We cannot have a truly authentic relationship with someone if we are unwilling or able to remove ourselves. Sometimes that means removing yourself a little ("Call me back when you are in a better mood.") or a lot ("I'm leaving.").

Here are some examples of how nice guys might communicate their boundaries assertively:

- "I am no longer willing to accept infidelity in our relationship. I expect honesty and respect from you moving forward, and if that is not something you can provide, I am open to discussing the possibility of separating."
- "I am happy to collaborate and contribute to team projects, but I need to set boundaries around my workload. I cannot take on additional projects now and must prioritize my commitments."
- "I value our friendship and enjoy spending

time together, but I also need time to myself. I will no longer be available to hang out every weekend, and I need to set aside time for my interests and hobbies."

By assertively communicating their boundaries, these Nice Guys can express their needs and wants clearly and respectfully while also setting limits and maintaining their own autonomy and well-being.

Here is how Ryan communicated his boundaries to his mother: "I love and respect you, Mom, but I need to set some boundaries around our relationship. I am an adult now and need to make decisions about my life. I understand that you have my best interests at heart, but I need to be able to make my own mistakes and learn from them. I hope you can respect my need for autonomy and support me in my decisions."

In this example, Ryan uses "I" statements to

express his feelings and is specific about his boundaries. He is also being firm but respectful in his communication and in expressing love and respect for his mother. By assertively communicating his boundaries, Ryan can establish a sense of respect and autonomy in his relationship with his mother while maintaining a positive and supportive dynamic.

Learning to Say "No"

Saying "no" is essential to setting and maintaining healthy boundaries in relationships. When we can say "no" to things that do not align with our values and limits, we can protect our well-being and establish a sense of respect and autonomy in our relationships.

Here are a few examples of the importance of saying "no" when setting boundaries:

- Protecting your physical well-being: Saying "no" to physical boundaries, such as setting limits around personal space or touch, can help protect your physical well-being and ensure that you feel safe and respected.

- Protecting your emotional well-being: Saying "no" to emotional boundaries, such as setting limits around how others can speak to you or what you are willing to share about yourself, can help protect your emotional well-being and ensure that you feel valued and respected.

- Setting limits around unhealthy behaviors: Saying "no" to unhealthy or disrespectful behaviors can help establish healthy boundaries in a relationship and ensure you are treated with respect.

Overall, saying "no" is essential to setting and maintaining healthy boundaries in relationships. By learning to assert your needs and wants and set limits with others, you can cultivate healthier, more fulfilling relationships and a more authentic sense of self.

Use only the necessary amount of resistance or strength when establishing boundaries.

When men first learn about setting boundaries, they tend to come on too strong. Dr. Glover refers to it as a "Kamikaze Boundary Setting." They expect a strong reaction and use excessive force when a more subtle approach suffices. Over time, they learn to use more finesse in their approach. People respond well to boundaries set by a strong, confident, calm individual who knows what he wants and expects. These boundaries are powerful but also kind, and people often appreciate them.

Neil Asserts His Boundaries

Neil realized that something had to change in his marriage as time passed. He decided to reclaim his masculinity and began seeking healthy role models and spending time with like-minded men. He started pursuing his passions and hobbies and even took up a few new ones. He began playing basketball with his friends, hiking in the mountains, and volunteering at a local animal shelter. These activities have helped him connect with other men, build self-confidence, and feel more fulfilled. He slowly became a more assertive and confident person, both in his personal and professional life.

But perhaps most importantly, he found the courage to set boundaries with his wife. He gave her an ultimatum, and while it was a difficult and emotional conversation, it ultimately led to his wife realizing the errors of her ways. She admitted to being impressed by and attracted to his assertiveness, and the two began couples counseling.

Summary

In conclusion, I will repeat how I started this

chapter. If someone continues to treat you badly, it's your fault. To stop tolerating someone's bad behavior is not just entirely in your control; it's your responsibility to yourself. When we don't take responsibility for our boundaries, we walk the world hiding and feeling scared.

Non-attachment to Outcome

"The more you know yourself, the more clarity there is. Self-knowledge has no end."

- Jiddu Krishnamurti

When you know yourself well, you can let go of your attachment to specific outcomes, because you're secure in your values and purpose. You're focused on the journey, not the destination, because you know that the journey is where growth and learning happen.

Recovering Nice Guys find themselves obsessing over the outcome of their actions, rather than focusing on the process itself. This attachment to outcome can prevent them from taking risks, trying new things, and ultimately living their best life. By cultivating non-attachment, they can learn to focus on the journey, rather than the destination.

Non-attachment means being focused on the process of your choosing, on one that aligns with your values and purpose, and not being attached to any specific outcome. When you're non-attached, you're open to learning and growing, and adjusting along the way. You're not concerned with whether you succeed or fail, but rather with the effort you put in and the experience you gain.

Non-attachment is not about being passive or indifferent; it's about being intentional and purposeful. When you're non-attached, you're not controlled by external circumstances, but rather by your own internal compass. You're able to navigate the twists and turns of life with ease, because you're not tied to any specific outcome.

You're focused on the present moment, and open to whatever comes your way.

So, in a way, non-attachment is about finding freedom within yourself. It's about cultivating a sense of inner peace and contentment that doesn't depend on external circumstances. When you're non-attached, you're free to live a life of purpose, fulfillment, and joy.

In the next chapter, we'll explore how to generate personal power. By focusing on your personal power, you can build the confidence and self-esteem you need to take risks and live the life you want. The next chapter will build on the concepts of non-attachment and help you take the next step on your journey to becoming a fully realized, integrated man.

After that, we'll move on to living in abundance. By cultivating a mindset of abundance, you can learn to see opportunities and possibilities where others see only obstacles. That chapter will help you shift your perspective from scarcity to abundance, and show you how to live a life of abundance in all areas of your life.

Generating Personal Power

What Is Personal Power?

Personal power is the ability to assert ourselves in the world and make choices that align with our values and goals. It is an internal, intrinsic source of power that comes from within and is not dependent on external factors such as status or wealth.

In contrast, external sources of power, such as status or wealth, are based on external factors and are often given to us by others. These sources of power can be fleeting and are not under our control.

Personal power can be cultivated through various means, including developing self-awareness, setting and maintaining healthy boundaries, building solid relationships, and taking ownership of our actions and decisions. By cultivating personal power, we can create positive change in our lives and relationships and live more authentic, fulfilling lives.

Personal power is the ability to take control of your own life and make the best decisions for *you*. It means standing up for yourself and asserting your own needs and desires, even in the face of challenges or obstacles. Personal power also involves setting healthy boundaries and being true to yourself rather than trying to please others or conform to their expectations. In short, personal power is about being the captain of your ship and navigating your way through life with confidence and intention.

Personal power is the ultimate hack for living a fulfilling and successful life. It's the key to breaking free from society's constraints and creating the kind of life you truly want. By developing your personal power, you'll be able to control your destiny and make the right choices rather than being a victim of circumstances. Whether you're looking to build a successful business, find the perfect romantic partner, or just be happy and fulfilled, personal power is the key to making it happen.

Here are the most common ways nice guys give away their power:

- By sacrificing their own needs and desires to please others
- By failing to set boundaries and allowing others to take advantage of their kindness
- By constantly seeking validation and approval from others
- By not standing up for themselves and allowing others to disrespect or mistreat them

- By not taking responsibility for their own actions and blaming others for their problems
- By being passive and not assertively pursuing their goals and aspirations
- By being overly accommodating and not asserting their own needs and desires in relationships
- By not taking care of their own physical and emotional well-being
- By not being honest and authentic with themselves and others

Limiting Beliefs that Take Away Personal Power

- Limiting beliefs are negative, self-defeating thoughts that hold us back and undermine our personal power. They can take the form of negative self-talk, such as "I am not good enough," or "I am not worthy," and can prevent us from taking action and pursuing our goals.

- Limiting beliefs often originate from past experiences or negative messages we receive from others, and they can become deeply ingrained in our thinking. They can be difficult to identify and challenge, but they can significantly impact our personal power and well-being.

- Limiting beliefs can cause a loss of personal power in several ways. For example, if we believe we are not good enough, we may be less likely to take risks or pursue our goals, as we are afraid of failure. This can prevent us from living our lives to the fullest and achieving our potential.

- Limiting beliefs can also cause us to undermine our own worth and value, leading us to accept treatment that is less than we deserve or to settle for less than we want in our lives.

- Overall, limiting beliefs can have a detrimental impact on our personal power and well-being. By identifying and challenging these beliefs, we can overcome them and cultivate a stronger, more authentic sense of self and the ability to assert ourselves in the world.

Here is a list of some of the most common limiting beliefs of Nice Guys:

- "I am not good enough."
- "I am not worthy of love or respect."
- "I am not deserving of happiness."
- "I am not capable of achieving my goals."
- "I have to put others' needs ahead of my own."
- "I have to be perfect to be accepted."
- "I am not strong enough to stand up for myself."
- "I don't deserve to have my own needs and wants."

- "I am not worthy of setting and maintaining healthy boundaries."
- "I am not deserving of respect or autonomy in my relationships."
- "I am not deserving of success or prosperity."
- "I am not capable of attracting and maintaining healthy relationships."
- "I am not capable of being my authentic self."
- "I am not worthy of having my own opinions or desires."
- "I have to do everything perfectly to be accepted."
- "I am not worthy of having my own boundaries or limits respected."
- "I am not capable of making my own decisions."
- "I am not deserving of having my own needs met."
- "I am not worthy of making my own choices."
- "I am not capable of being independent or

self-sufficient."

Taking Back Your Personal Power

If you're a nice guy who feels like you've been giving away your power, it's time to take control and get it back.

Identify the areas where you tend to give your power away. This might be in your relationships, career, or personal life. Take some time to think about where you feel most powerless.

Make a list of ways you can take back your power in these areas. This might include setting boundaries, practicing assertiveness, or finding ways to feel more confident and self-assured.

Choose a few strategies from your list that feel doable and meaningful to you. Try to tackle only some things at first – pick a few to focus on and work on those.

Put your chosen strategies into action. This might mean saying "no" to unreasonable requests, speaking up for yourself, or finding ways to take care of yourself.

Celebrate your progress and continue to work on building your personal power. Remember that this is a process; it takes time and effort to reclaim your power.

Here are some more practical ways to start getting your personal power back:

- Practice gratitude and focus on the positive things in your life.
- Set clear goals and take action toward achieving them.
- Cultivate healthy relationships and surround yourself with supportive people.
- Take care of your physical and mental health through self-care practices like exercise, meditation, and coaching.

- Embrace your quirks and uniqueness.

- Practice assertiveness and set boundaries with others.

- Build a strong sense of self-worth and confidence by building your competence.

- Find your passion and pursue it with enthusiasm.

- Take control of your finances and manage your resources effectively.

Neil Reclaims His Personal Power

Neil used to be passive-aggressive, always trying to please his wife and avoid conflict. But deep down, he was resentful and unhappy. One day, he had had enough. He decided to take control of his life and get his personal power back.

First, he set some boundaries with his wife. He told her he wouldn't tolerate her rude behavior anymore and expect to be treated with respect. To his surprise, his wife appreciated his assertiveness, and things started to improve in their relationship.

Neil also discovered some new passions and hobbies in his 40s. He started playing the guitar and even joined a band. He also took up skydiving and became an adrenaline junkie. His newfound confidence and zest for life made him more attractive to his wife.

In addition to finding new hobbies, he also took control of his finances. He drew a line with his wife about household expenses and started managing their money more effectively. This helped to reduce a lot of the stress and tension in their marriage.

Neil's journey to getting his personal power back was bumpy, but it was worth it. He learned to be more assertive, set boundaries, and pursue his passions. And as a result, his marriage improved, and he became a happier, more fulfilled person.

Ryan Becomes True to Himself

Ryan realized that living his life for girls' approval was not fulfilling, and he was not living up to his true potential. He made a decision to reclaim his personal power.

He started by working on building his social skills. He went out more and clarified his intentions when talking to people, especially girls. He stopped worrying about what they would think of him and instead focused on being himself. This new assertive attitude made him more confident and attractive.

Ryan also focused on his physical well-being. He started exercising regularly, which gave him a clear head and a sense of discipline. The discipline of the exercise regimen began spilling into other areas of his life.

As he worked on himself, he realized that taking care of himself was the key to true happiness. He stopped seeking validation from others and instead focused on living his life on his own terms. He made decisions that were true to himself and that made him happy.

Ryan discovered that as he focused less on seeking validation from others and more on being true to himself, he began to attract people to him. His newfound confidence and assertiveness were paying off.

Confidence Is a Result, Not an Entitlement

Everybody wants confidence before they begin something new, but it's the payoff for taking action when you feel afraid. Fear is often a mask for desire, which means your lack of confidence becomes your compass, quietly pointing you in the direction of what you really want to do.

Personal power, therefore, is a result of our decision and subsequent actions to stand up for ourselves. We cannot wait to reclaim our personal power when we have confidence. Instead, in the process of taking courageous action, we build personal power and confidence.

Living In Abundance

As we navigate life, getting caught up in our own problems and challenges is easy. We often focus on what we don't have rather than the abundance surrounding us. But when we take a step back and really look at our lives, it's clear that we are incredibly fortunate. We have access to an abundance of love, beauty, and opportunity.

Let's start with the simple things that we often take for granted. The warmth of the sun on our skin, the cool breeze in our hair, the sound of birds singing in the morning. These are all examples of the abundance of nature that surrounds us daily. The world is full of breathtaking landscapes and natural wonders that remind us of the beauty and majesty of the earth.

Next, there's the abundance of love in our lives. The love of our family, friends, and loved ones is a constant source of support and joy. A simple hug or a kind word can make all the difference in the world. Even in the darkest of times, we can find solace and comfort in the love of those around us.

We also have an abundance of opportunities and possibilities. We live in an age where we can access knowledge, resources, and technology to help us achieve our dreams and goals. We can pursue our passions and make a difference in the world.

Despite our challenges and struggles, we are incredibly fortunate to be alive. We have the opportunity to experience the world's beauty and wonder, love and be loved, and make our mark on the planet. We are surrounded by abundance, and it's up to us to open our eyes and hearts to see it.

Nice Guys and the Scarcity Mindset

Nice guys often have a scarcity mindset. They believe that love, respect, and acceptance are limited resources that they must compete for. They see the world as a zero-sum game where if someone else wins, they must lose. This mentality leads them to believe that if anyone else is in a relationship, there must be something wrong with them. They see the world as a cold, uncaring place where they must fight for every scrap of affection they receive.

This mentality is not entirely their fault. It is often the result of societal conditioning and past experiences that have taught them that they are not enough and must strive to earn love and acceptance. They have been taught that they must be perfect, be everything to everyone, and always put others' needs before their own.

But there are more fulfilling ways to move through the world than living with a scarce mentality. It leads to feelings of inadequacy, resentment, and despair. A more fulfilling way of living is to build the ability to see and enjoy the abundance around us. An abundant mentality is one where we believe there is enough love, respect, and acceptance to go around. It's a belief that we are enough and deserve to be loved and respected for who we are.

As I said at the start of the book, being nice is not a bad thing. Being kind, compassionate, and caring matters. But it's about doing it without a hidden agenda. It's about learning to put ourselves first, set healthy boundaries, and believe that we are worthy of love and respect. It's about learning to see the world as a place of abundance, where there is enough for everyone.

Developing an Abundance Mindset

Developing a gratitude practice and an abundance mindset can seem daunting, but it doesn't have to be. In fact, it can be a fun and rewarding experience. Here are some simple ways to get started.

- Keep a gratitude journal. Each day, take a few minutes to write down three things you're grateful for. Reflecting on the good things in our lives helps shift our focus from what we lack to what we have. Pro-tip: Find someone with whom you can share this list daily.
- Practice mindfulness. Take a moment each day to be present in the moment. Whether

through meditation, yoga, or simply walking outside, mindfulness helps us appreciate the beauty and abundance in our lives.

- Surround yourself with positive people. The people we surround ourselves with have a significant impact on our mindset. Surround yourself with people with an abundant mindset who are positive and supportive.

- Give back. Helping others is a powerful way to shift our focus from our struggles to the world's abundance.

- Make it fun! Gratitude and abundance are not about being serious all the time. Make it fun and light-hearted, and enjoy the process.

This is not a one-time fix but a way of being. Be kind and patient with yourself, and remember that small steps lead to significant changes.

Epilogue

As we come to the end of this book, I want to reflect on the journey that Ryan, Rowan, and Neil have taken. While these characters are semi-fictional, they are indeed a combination of all the nice guys I have coached and my own story.

It would be easy to say that Ryan, Rowan, and Neil went on to have the perfect life after their journey of Nice Guy recovery. But life doesn't work that way. Life is a splendid kaleidoscope of ups and downs, sweat and tears, victories and defeats. As recovering Nice Guys, it's easy to get caught up in pursuing a non-existent perfect future while ignoring the beauty and abundance of all that we already have and all that is already lovable about us. Our work is to learn to embrace our imperfections and the glorious uncertainties of life and recognize that we grow through these challenges. Let's be proud of our progress and the person we're becoming daily.

The book's introduction explored the importance of male initiation in the Nice Guy recovery work. The process of initiating men into their true selves is powerful and transformative. It's a journey that involves facing our fears, embracing our vulnerabilities, and taking responsibility for our leadership. It's not always easy, but it is incredibly rewarding.

As men, we often struggle with feeling like we have to have it all figured out. We're taught to be strong, confident, and in control at all times. But the truth is, we all have moments of doubt and insecurity. And that's okay. The Nice Guy recovery work is about embracing those moments and using them as opportunities for growth and self-discovery.

I encourage you to take the journey. It may be challenging, but it is so worth it. When men take responsibility for their leadership, they not only transform their own lives but also positively impact the world around them. They become role models for other men and for the next generation.

As you progress in your journey, remember that you are not alone. There is a community of men who are on this journey with you. Lean on each other, support each other, and hold each other accountable. Together, we can make the world a better place.

Thank you for taking the time to read this book. I hope that you've found it helpful and that it has given you the tools and inspiration to begin your journey of Nice Guy recovery. Remember, you are worthy of love, respect, and acceptance. You deserve to live a fulfilling and authentic life. I believe in you. The world is waiting for you to step into your greatness.

About the Author

Sidharth is obsessed with supporting men in recovering from their Nice Guy syndrome, and becoming integrated, emotionally and physically healthy, and getting on-purpose in their lives. He is also the founder of *ManKind Project India*.

He is a lifelong educator with a fierce passion to help people realize their full human potential. As a certified No More Mr. Nice Guy coach and a leadership development coach, he has led workshops around the world. He brings a unique combination of modalities to his work which include Mindfulness, Co-active Coaching, Non-violent Communication, Radical Honesty, Conscious Leadership and Yoga. He leads contemplative leadership journeys to the Everest

Basecamp twice a year. He is an avid Vipassana meditator. Visit wildmancoaching.com for one-on-one and group coaching.

Made in the USA
Monee, IL
10 June 2025

19190375R00105